I0447443

Anal Sex Tips
For Guys and Girls

By

Angelicka Wallows

Edited by Angelicka Wallows

DISCLAIMER

This publication is meant to offer informative material only. It is sold with the understanding that its contributors are not offering professional service or advice. For any health conditions or questions, you should consult a health professional to diagnose and treat that condition and answer your questions. Before copying any activity described herein, such as giving or receiving anal sex, the reader should consult a competent professional for advice.

While the publisher and author have done their best in preparing this book, they make no representation or warranty regarding its contents, and specifically disclaim any implied warranties for any particular purpose. The publisher also assumes no responsibility for errors or omissions, and assumes no liability for damages resulting from the use of information or ideas herein or from following acts described herein. The fact that a person, organization, article or website may be referred to herein as a citation or a possible source of information does not mean that the publisher endorses such sources, their information or their recommendations.

Readers should consult an appropriate professional for all physical, mental or health conditions, treatments or questions related to this topic.

CONTENTS

FOREWORD

I have always been interested in trying new sorts of pleasures, and obviously anal sex is one of them. I admit that I started quite early and got the chance to do it with two great partners the first time, which made me enjoy it right away. As I am getting a lot of questions about it on my blog, I decided to share my few years experience on the matter with you, as well as the testimonials I got from many readers.

When done right, anal sex is extremely pleasurable, and a delicious way to spice up and diversify your sexual life. So why not give it a try?

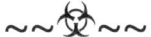

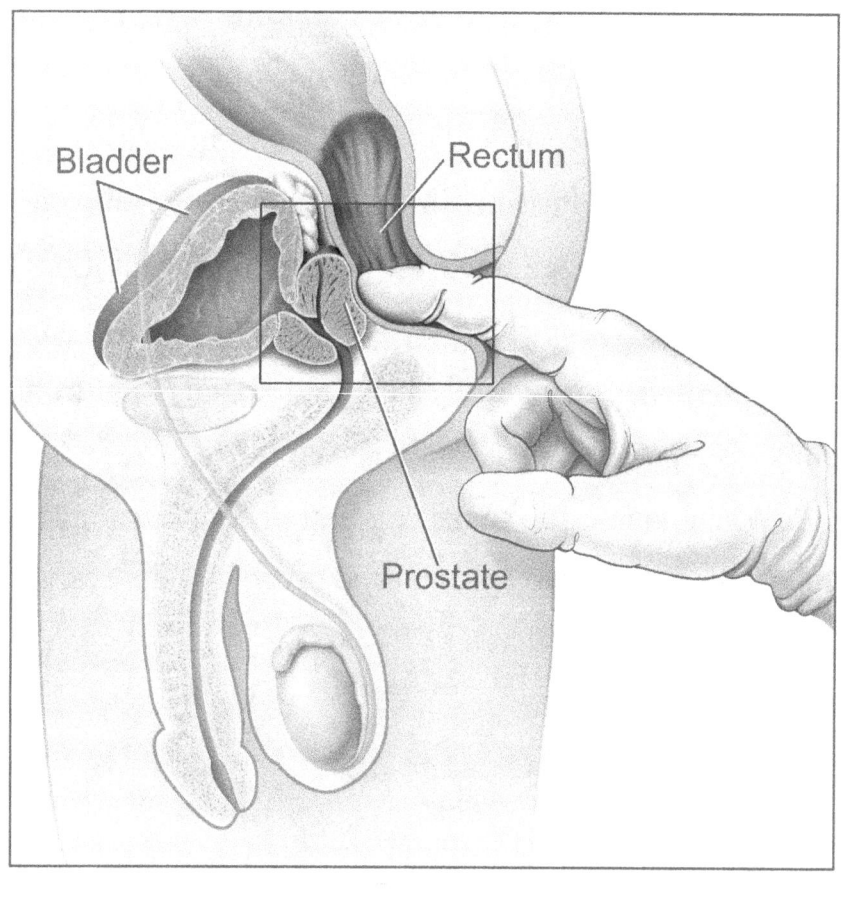

1/ UNDERSTANDING THE RECTUM

A little bit of anatomy here guys! If you've got to stick your penis somewhere, you'd better understand how it is configured so that you know how to actually get it in.

Unlike the vagina, the anus is not a straight path. It is more like an "S" shaped path. The entry of this path is guarded by two strong muscles: the internal and external anal sphincters. It is the contraction of these muscles that causes pain during anal penetration, and it is their relaxation that makes it a pleasurable act. The rule here is to keep them relaxed. You can achieve that by good preparation, generous lubrication, and by "pushing" gently, just like you do when you defecate (which is why I like to deep clean myself first, as it boosts my confidence in doing so). Pushing when you try to get a penis inside is can seem a bit contradictory (and that's probably why it is said to be against nature!), but doing so will tremendously facilitate the penetration. You can practice Kegel exercises, just like you do with your vagina, to master anal relaxation and become more aware of your backside.

The first sphincter is fairly easy to pass, but the second one is a bit harder, so just take your time, go bit by bit, relax, pull out and start again. Once you managed to pass it, that's it! That's where the pleasure starts!

After the sphincters, the rectum takes an upward curve. So guys, once you popped open her pleasure hole, don't just dive straight in! If your cock is straight, bear in mind that curve and give your penetration a bit of drift upwards. If your cock is more like the curvy kind, then penetrate your partner so that the curve of your tool follows the curve of his or her rectum.

A little bit deeper in, the rectum will make another gentle curve. These curves have to be dealt with carefully. Don't fuck her hard like you would do to her pussy, because that really hurts. Take the time to both explore and discover the different sensations. Being conscious of your own body and of your partner's body will drastically increase your pleasure, not only for anal sex, but for your sex life in general. Anal is a great way to discover each other's body as well as your own, because of the special attention you need to put into it.

After a while, once you two really master the art of sodomy, you will be able to add strength and depth to the act, but to start with, just be gentle.

~~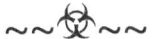~~

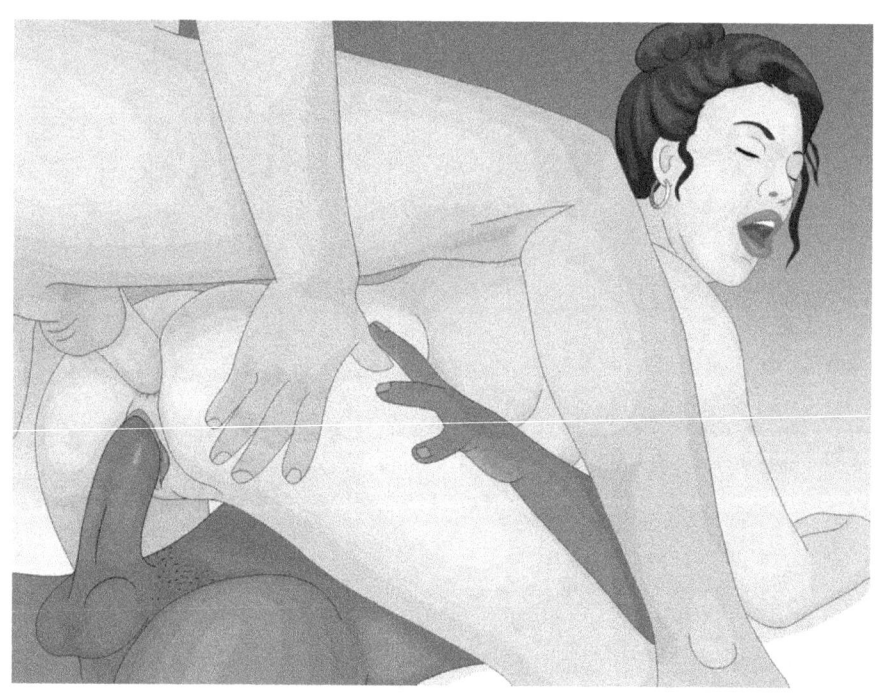

2/ TALK ABOUT IT WITH YOUR PARTNER(S)

Anal sex is a taboo for many. Deciding to go for it is already a great step, but it is important that you have a serious conversation with your partner(s) about it. I say partner(s) here because my first anal experience was with 2 guys. It was really awesome because one of them was really making me feel relaxed and hungry for it, while the other was taking the virginity of my little pink ass. I am not saying here that you should engage in a threesome for the sake of having your anus deflowered. Hell no! Follow your own sexual preferences! But whoever is involved in this first time, get together and talk. What should you talk about?

Well, about the limits: set the rules of the game. The one who is penetrated must have full power, and they are the one to decide when to stop, or when to continue. This will not only help the penetrated person be more confident, and therefore more able to relax, but will also draw the boundaries for all parties involved. Talk about what you want to experiment with, talk about the long preliminaries you want to have and how you want to have them. Make sure you prepare in advance and that you don't rush things.

Then again, talk during the act. Whenever it feels good, express it. If it starts to hurt a little, gently pull out a bit and let your partner know. Guide his/her way to your pleasure. Use your vocal command to drive his cock into your tight hole the way it feels better for you. Experiment different paces, different angles, different depth, and let him know each time how it feels. Educate your penetrator to your likes.

Once the climax has been reached, whether you managed to be anally deflowered or not, take the time to talk about it again with your partner(s). Describe your experience, your fears, your turn-ons... Share those little details that make a big difference so that next time you indulge in buggery, you can increase your level of mastery.

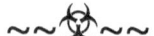

3/ KEEP IT CLEAN

Unless you are constipated, your anal area doesn't usually keep any feces. It is important to understand how your digestive system works; you see, from the moment you ingest food until the moment you defecate, the food follows a certain process that will transfer its nutrients and energy to your body. It is transported by muscular contractions in your bowels, not by gravity, and these contractions follow a cycle. Once you have expelled the unused matter, it will take another cycle before more waste comes all the way down meters of intestine inside you. Well, that's kind of common sense but it doesn't hurt to clarify.

Even though you are naturally "clean" inside after you defecated, some like to perform extra cleanup before going for an anal intercourse. It is actually a good practice, not only because you can enjoy even cleaner sex, but also because it improves your metabolism and has a positive impact on your body, such as helping you with constipation, bad breath, weight problems, indigestion, preventing flatulence, and more.

*

Bowel cleansing, also called an "enema," can be performed two ways: orally and anally.

Oral enema:

It is recommended that you do it when you wake up in the morning, or a few hours before engaging into anal sex. Here is how to prepare it: add two level teaspoons of uniodized sea salt (regular or iodized salt will not have the same beneficial effect) to a liter of lukewarm water. Shake well, and then drink the entire liter at once. It's also good to massage the colon as well. This oral enema will flush out your entire digestive tract and colon from top to bottom, usually within an hour, prompting you to eliminate several times, clearing out the plaque and debris from the walls, and the parasites that have been living there. The quantity of salt is important, as it is meant to give the water the same density as your blood.

Anal enema:

There are different sorts of anal enemas. The most commonly used (which I find to be the best in my case), would be a douche bag (about 2 liters), a soft tube, and a nozzle. Other kinds of enema equipment exist, such as a nozzle that you can adapt to your shower hose, a pear-shape rectal bulb syringe, or some more complex apparatus. You can also use different sorts of mixtures to inject in your rectum, depending on the result you want to achieve (herbal concoction, coffee, lemon, and more). I will not develop the subject further here, as it is not the purpose of this guide, but you can definitely find a lot more details on the internet, or you may simply want to buy a book on the subject (The New Detox Bath is a good title to read to start getting familiar with enema, as is Enema Guide).

*

OK, now that I have told you a bit about enemas, you should know that not only it will have a positive impact on your body, but also it will help you get more relaxed before penetration. Knowing that your sphincter is clean will help you relax more and give the little "push" that will open it for penetration.

Also one thing that adds comfort to the act: keep your crack smooth and free of hair! Yes, get rid of the hair in your anal area! If you can't afford waxing or going to the salon to have someone remove your hair around there, then either shave it yourself with a razor or use a hair removal cream, which is usually quite efficient (test it for skin allergy first though). I personally don't like shaving. My skin is sensitive, and shaving always leaves me with a reddish bump after a couple of days, which is neither nice nor comfortable.

Being smooth and clean is always a big plus in anal intercourse!

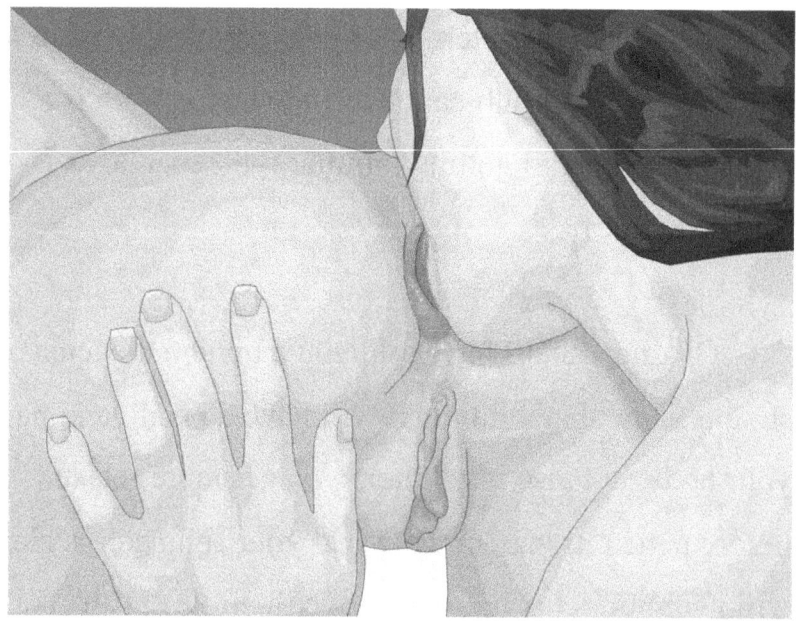

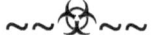

4/ GET IT READY

Preliminaries are even more important for anal sex than for vaginal sex. The purpose here is to make your partner relaxed enough to accept anal penetration, and physically prepare the anus to be popped.

Rimming is a must. Don't forget that, if you followed my advice up to here, your partner would be thoroughly clean, inside out. So licking that little hole shouldn't turn you off. On the contrary! The anal area is full of nerves and very sensitive. It is probably one of the most erogenous zones of the body. Playing with the anus is teasing like hell. You can decide to perform a gently massage, lick it passionately with your tongue, or caress it with a feather. Let your imagination run wild and experiment with new things with your partner. You will gradually witness that the anus starts to open up like a cute little pink flower. That's a sign that your partner has started to really relax and that you are on the right path.

But don't jump in at the first occasion; make your playmate long for it! Continue your teasing and start preparing the back door. It is a good idea to progressively lubricate it, making it part of the foreplay. Gently insert some KY jelly (or any water based lube) into the pooper with your finger. When you do so, make sure that your fingers are well manicured and that you carefully cleaned them before, out of respect for your partner. This will allow your brown eye to slightly open up. Again the rule is not to force-penetrate it. Be gentle and let it absorb your finger. If your partner is up to it, you may want to try a second finger, or maybe use a small size dildo or a butt plug. Make it last and gradually increase the grid and the depth of the insertions, until you get to something that matches the size of your cock. Well, that may not happen all at once, and it could take a few sessions before your partner can accept something of the size of your dick, especially if you are well endowed.

Let me open just a parenthesis here for something very important: you can always go from pussy to ass, but NEVER from ass to pussy. Be it your cock, fingers, dildo, cucumber, you name it! If you use condoms, remove the condom you used for her ass and put on a new one to fuck her vagina. No matter how much you cleaned your rectum, this is just not compatible. A quick tip here is to keep within reach of your hand one of those travel hand sanitizers (the rinse-free ones work wonders) as well as sanitizing wipes.

Don't insert anything that could break, split, cut or harm the anus in any way. This is a very sensitive area, exposed to germs on a regular basis, and not easy to heal. Should you want to experiment with fruits and vegetables, always wash them thoroughly with a small concentration of bleach, and then with some vinegar. Rinse, dry, and cover them with a condom. If you use toys, always make sure to disinfect them before and after use. When you want to play real dirty, it is a must to have irreproachable hygiene. You can find a lot of fun toys to play with, as well as diverse accessories and lubes on Amazon.com.

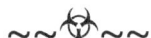

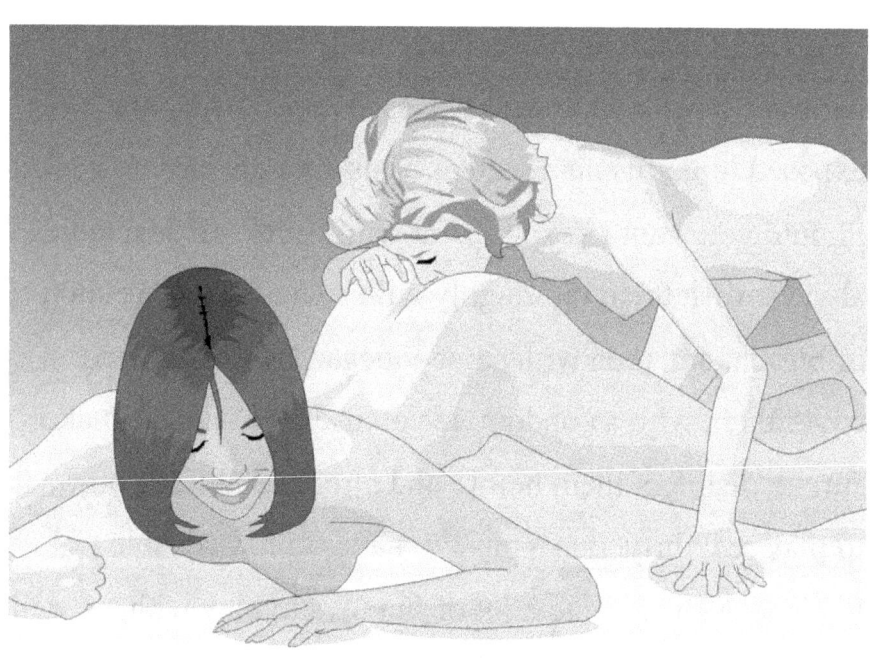

5/ LUBE IT BABY!

Relaxation and lubrication are the two pillars of anal penetration. The previous steps focused mainly on relaxation,

A water based lube is a must. Oil-based lube would damage the latex of the condom or the toys you are using, so keep away from it. Talking about condoms, it is a must if you engage into anal sex with casual partners. Barebacking may sound fun, but be aware that anal intercourse, when unprotected, is an open door for STD. Not only is the rectum fragile and able to easily be damaged, but it also hosts a lot of different bacteria, no matter how well you clean it beforehand. Be thoughtful of your partner and of yourself.

Back to the lube. As you know, the anal region is not naturally lubricated. Adding a lot of lube is therefore an absolute necessity. However, the thing about water-based lube is that it tends to dry up more quickly than oil-based lubes. You can easily "reactivate" it, however, by adding a bit more lube (or water, or saliva) every now and then, to keep it slippery and wet. Also avoid flavored lubes. They can sometimes irritate the skin and are not really meant to be used for anal penetration, as they often are for external use only.

You may also use silicone-based lubes. They last longer than water-based lubes, however, they have the tendency to damage toys made of silicone. They are also harder to wash off, and may cause some irritation. It is a good idea to test it first and see how comfortable you feel with it. For your information, please note that Vaseline is an oil-based lube, and therefore shouldn't be used for sexual intercourse.

For those interested, I have run into a natural homemade lube. Here is the recipe:

Mix and heat 4 table spoons of cornstarch and 1 cup of water until completely dissolved in a covered saucepan. Use non-metallic dishes and a non-metallic stirring spoon. Cool it down. Pour some into a dispenser bottle. Refrigerate remainder.

I confess I haven't tried it, so if you want to give it a try, do it at your own risk.

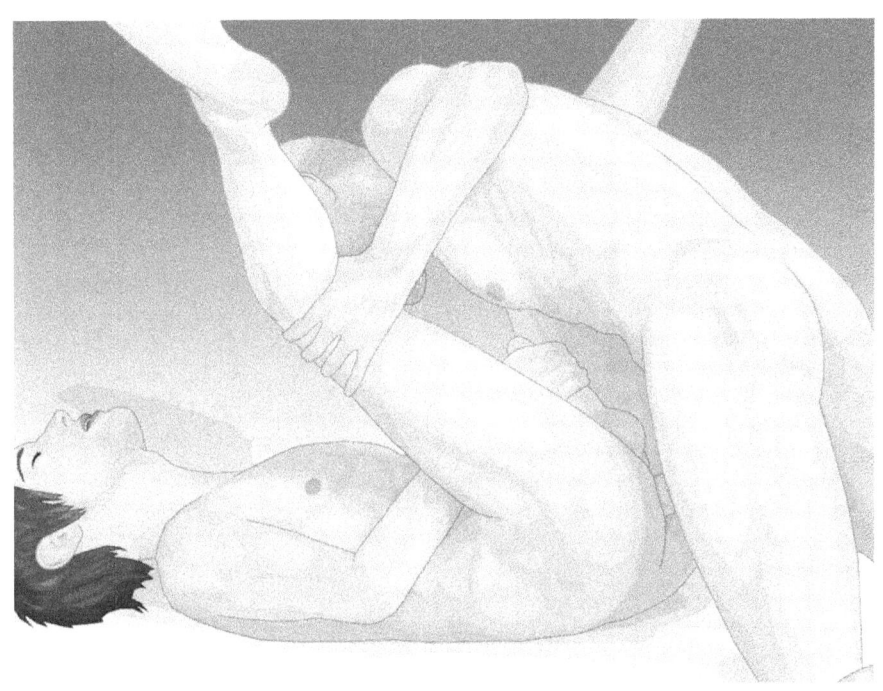

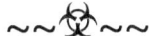

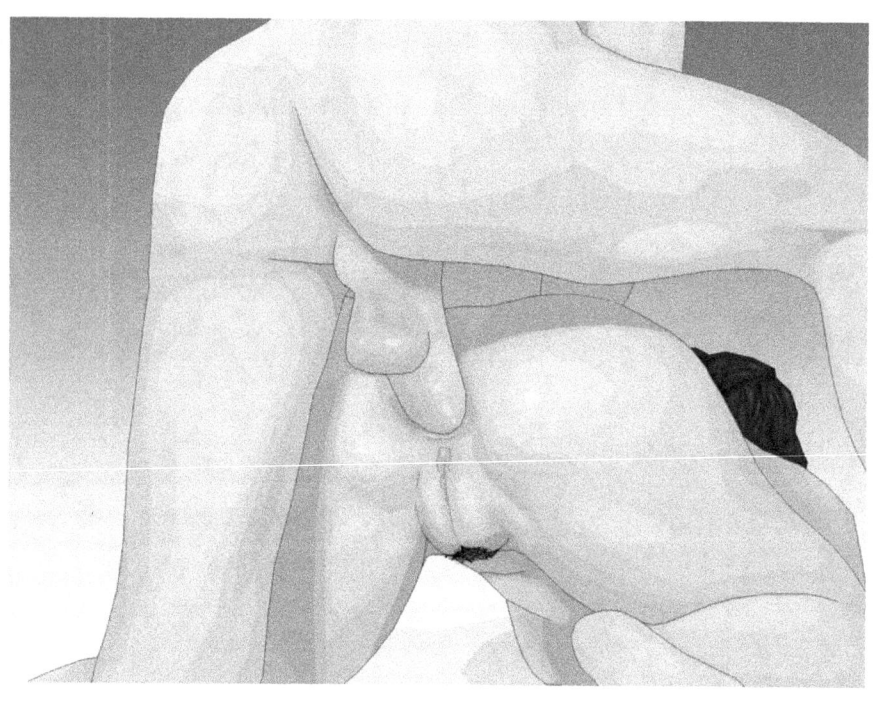

6/ PENETRATION

Here you are! The anus is ready to be deflowered! Congratulations! But hey! How should you start?

Well, actually there are two options here:

The first option is that the penetrated person takes the lead and rides the cock. That means that the girl (or guy) would eventually sit on her partner's cock, most probably in the cowgirl position. Talking about the penetrated point of view, this position lets you be in control of everything, and do whatever you want, when and how you want it. However, your body posture may not be appropriate for an optimum anal penetration. A sitting position would accentuate the curves of your rectum (as we have seen in the Chapter 1 of this book), making it more difficult to penetrate.

The other position you can go with is the reverse missionary (where the penetrated person lays on her tummy). You can even place a pillow under your pubis to adjust the angle of penetration. I definitely find this position more comfortable; you can completely relax that way, be more receptive, and enjoy it more! But if you choose this option, make it very clear that when you say stop, he should stop. Well, make it very clear that your partner should obey you instantly, whatever you tell him or her. Talk to your penetrator and guide him, and don't let him be adventurous on your first time.

Leave the other positions (such as doggie style) to the experienced sodomites.

Now that your partner is well lubed and ready to take it in the ass, make sure that you listen to your partner, and that you go extremely slowly. The hardest part will be to pass the head of your cock through the two sphincters, but if you followed the steps of this guide, it should happen seamlessly. Once you are in there, don't push in the full length of your dick. Give your partner half of it for a start; this will be more than enough. Once you are inside, stop and let your partner relax, and her anus adjust to your girth. This moment provides great sensations to the penetrator, and gives a feeling of domination and power, while the penetrated feels (and is) at the mercy of her partner.

Once adjusted, try to do a few ins and outs, again very slowly. Then I would recommend that you pull out (still very slowly) if it is your first time. For the more experienced ass fuckers, you can go deeper and a bit faster, but always hold your horses unless your partner begs you to go harder. Once you have been opened, you can experience different positions and see which one gives you the most pleasure.

In any case, after penetrating an ass hole, always remove your condom and clean your cock. Whatever was in an ass shouldn't go anywhere else until it has been thoroughly cleaned.

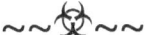

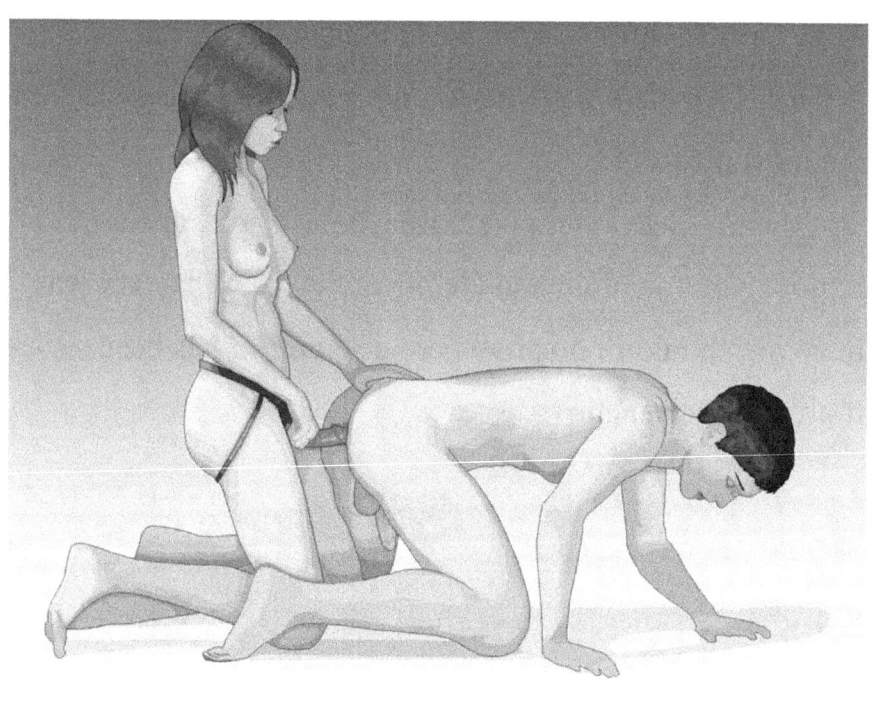

7/ TOYS STORIES

Toys are part of the anal sex fun, and there are quite a lot available on the market, to enjoy solo or with your partner(s). Now the same rules apply for toys:

1) Whatever comes out of an ass must be disinfected

2) Use lots of lube

3) Penetrate very slowly

4) Listen to your partner

*

Here are a few descriptions of the most common anal toys (source: Wikipedia):

Anal plugs

A butt plug is a sex toy designed to be inserted in the anus and rectum for sexual pleasure. In some ways, they are similar to a dildo, but they tend to be shorter, and must have a flanged end to prevent the device from being lost inside the rectum. They are primarily worn for a short period of time to prepare the anus for anal sex, stretching and relaxing the sphincter muscles to comfortably accept a penis or other penetrative device.

Anal beads

Anal beads are a sex toy consisting of multiple spheres or balls linked together in series which are continuously inserted through the anus into the rectum and then removed with varying speeds depending on the effect desired (most typically during the orgasm, to enhance climax). Those who use anal beads enjoy the pleasurable feeling they receive as the ball passes through the narrow sphincter of the anus.

Dildo

A dildo is a sex toy, often explicitly phallic in appearance, intended for bodily penetration during masturbation or sex with partners.

Strap-on Dildo

A strap-on dildo (also strap-on, dildo harness) is a dildo designed to be worn, usually with a harness, during sexual activity. Harnesses and dildos are made in a wide variety of styles, with variations in how the harness fits the wearer, how the dildo attaches to the harness, as well as various features intended to facilitate stimulation of the wearer or a sexual partner.

A strap-on dildo can be used for a wide variety of sexual activities, including solo or mutual masturbation, as well as penetrative oral, anal, or vaginal sex. Strap-on dildos can be used by people of any sexuality or gender, and upon people of any sexuality or gender.

Vibrator

Vibrators are devices for the body and skin, to stimulate the nerves for a relaxing and pleasurable feeling. Some vibrators are designed to ergonomically stimulate erogenous zones for erotic stimulation.

*

Using toys can be a great way to prepare and educate yourself on the pleasures of anal penetration. It is highly recommended to use proper toys, especially for beginners. It makes a sound investment to buy one in a sex shop (or even online). I usually do my sex toys shopping online with Eden Fantasy's, as they have a great choice of really cool toys, but you are really free to buy wherever you like.

Always make sure to disinfect your toys BEFORE and AFTER use. Store them clean and dry, away from direct sunlight. And remember: never use oil-based lube with your toys, as it would damage them.

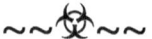

IN CONCLUSION

Anal sex should now be demystified. You may or may not want to try it. If you go for it, make sure it is of your own free will, and do your research first. I have been practicing anal sex for years now and I must confess that I love it. With time and practice, you can tolerate larger cocks or dildos, and can still enjoy the slight pain of the first penetration, that soon changes into an incredible source of pleasure.

Should you have any question, please feel free to contact me through my website and I will be more than happy to answer you to the best of my knowledge.

Remember, it is important to always practice safe sex: don't put yourself or your partner at risk!

###

ABOUT THE AUTHOR

Angelicka Wallows is a young, mysterious, and posh girl who likes to have a good time and to live life to the fullest.
She likes the outdoors, has a secret collection of toys, and loves to spread her wings and discover new horizons!
She enjoys letting her hair down and feel the breeze caressing her bare skin.
Angelicka holds a Master in Business Administration but that doesn't mean that she is all books! After her long working day managing a large corporation, she swaps her corporate suit for sexy lingerie, and dives in her secret universe: Erotica.

www.ingramcontent.com/pod-product-compliance
Lightning Source LLC
Chambersburg PA
CBHW072223290526
45794CB00007B/2869